ROCK YOUR BODY

AND

THE PLANET

Little changes can make a big difference

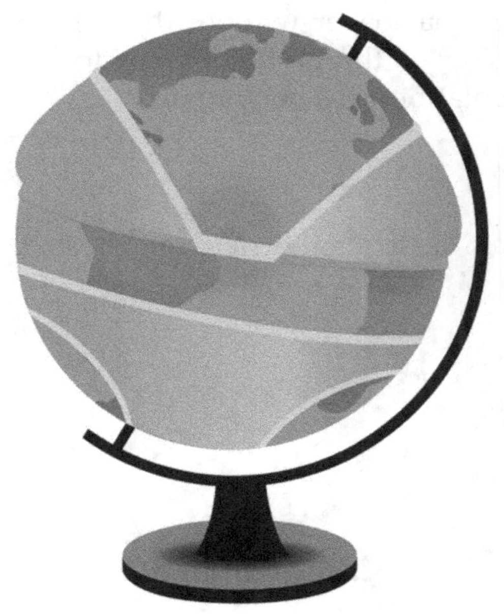

BARBARA HANNAH

Cover art illustration by Aubrey Shearer

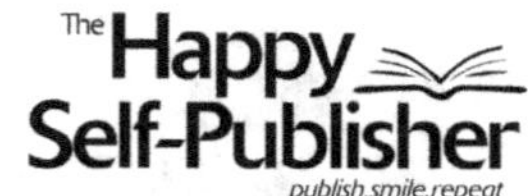

www.happyselfpublisher.com

ACKOWLEDGMENTS

Thank you to the people in the corporate office whose directive resulted in my second college degree. Thank you to my manager at the time, Chris, who accepted my proposal and allowed me to enroll. Thank you to my next manager, Lori, who allowed me to continue on the path that I had started with Chris. Thank you to my family, especially my mom. I lost her to cancer not even a year after she sat in the stadium and watched me walk to get my second college degree. Thank you to the other moms I talked to at my kids' events, who suggested that I write a book. Thank you to Lois for holding the writing workshop that gave me the tools I needed to turn my idea into the work that you are about to read, and to Dana for making my thoughts easy to read. Thank you to the staff and professors at the University of Delaware College of Earth, Ocean and Environment for being awesome and doing the work that you do, especially Frank, who was assistant dean at the time that I enrolled. His support in my plan was instrumental.

INTRODUCTION

One day while I was sitting in traffic, it occurred to me that the kinds of things the environmentalists are touting as the right things to do for the earth were pretty much the same things I'd been reading about in fitness books and magazines.

I was in my early 40s at the time, and a single mother of three active kids. Driving kids around all the time, while exhausting, does not count as aerobic activity and I was showing the signs of a 40-something-year-old woman who sat too much. I spent my days at work sitting in an office chair and my evenings driving my kids around. My typical day looked like this -- get up, make lunches, make coffee, get the kids up and ready, take them to school, go to work, drive home, make dinner, drive to sports practice, homework (the order depended upon the day of the week), then showers and bed.

I care about the environment. I care about my physical fitness. But, just how the heck was I supposed to take action on either one? I really hadn't seen any practical advice that could work for me. I know myself. I'm not going to do things like drink cabbage juice and I spend my lunch hour running errands.

My daily routine made my life full; but then, it got fuller. Someone in the corporate office decided that everyone with my job description needed to have a science degree. This was bad news. I had a degree in marketing, and although it was a bachelor of science, by no stretch of the imagination was that a science degree. The deck seemed to be stacked against me as a single mom with no savings outside of my 401K. Even though I had been doing the job

– and doing it well – for more than four years, if I wanted to keep it, I needed to take action.

I glanced at the website of the local university (University of Delaware) and saw the College of Earth Ocean and Environment had a degree in environmental studies with a concentration in environmental law, policy and politics. Perfect! I've always loved the ocean. I convinced my boss that this degree at UD was relevant to my job and would meet the "science degree" requirement. He approved my enrollment under my company's tuition reimbursement plan. I applied and was accepted at UD and added "part-time college student" to my already busy life. I had to get creative with my scheduling, but I made it work. Along the way I figured out how to do things to benefit both the planet and my body simultaneously.

Most people have the motivation to heal their bodies and the planet but fail to take action because they don't know where to start. Every time I've shared some of these ideas, someone suggests that I should write a book, so I did! We only get one body, and we've only got one planet. So, if you are interested in some practical things that you can do to rock your body and the planet, then listen up. My goal is to help you turn your thoughts into actions and empower you to go after your goals.

MOVE YOUR BODY

When I talk about physical fitness, I am talking about what you do with your body. Many people equate physical fitness with working out at the gym. I hate going to the gym. It's not that I've had bad experiences at the gym. I just don't enjoy working out there. It was always the same. Do so many of these. Work this then work that. Yeah, yeah, yeah, okay. If you love the gym, that's great – keep at it. If you don't love it – it's OK, just do something else. You have lots of other options to move your body.

Choose a sport

If you're like me and you read fitness books and magazines, you might have seen the advice to join a sport. Well, Taxi-Mom isn't really a sport, although there are enough of us to form a national league. So how are you supposed to join a sport? If you are sporty and can join a local adult league for something, that's great. The general rule is that if you find a sport that you enjoy, you are more likely to stick with it, and maybe even have fun! If you try and force yourself to do something that you don't enjoy then you won't stick with it.

Take a walk

So, what do you do if there aren't any local sports or leagues you like or the ones available don't fit into your schedule? Walking is good, if you are able. I have a smart-watch device that tracks my steps. Every little bit helps.

The environmentalists will tell you to drive less and walk more. Well, I hear you enviros; but for a Mom in the suburbs with kids in travel sports, the concept of drive less and walk more is not practical. I keep my tires full and get good gas mileage, but that is the best that I can do with my driving impact on the environment.

You have to be creative. I see some parents doing laps around the building where my son practices gymnastics. If the sports complex where your kid practices has stairs, then take a few trips up and down the stairs during practice.

I find a walk can give me some nice alone time when I'm able to fit one in. I'm often challenged by feelings of guilt when I'm walking, because I feel I should be doing something "more important." It takes practice and persistence to keep from falling victim to that. One approach is to sign up for a walk for charity. Websites like Races2Run.com list all the walks and runs that are coming up complete with links to sign up right on line. Who can argue with walking for a good cause?

Walk a dog

Do you have a dog? Maybe your neighbor's dog would like to get out more often. If not, there are plenty of dogs in the local animal shelter that would love for you to come walk them and play with them. Animal shelter volunteer dog walker is a thing – check it out.

State Parks

Not into dogs? Do you like nature? There are state parks with trails waiting to be explored. Trails to walk, hike, or ride a bike. Some of my local state parks have ponds where you can take out a canoe, kayak, row boat, or SUP (stand up paddleboard). You are getting exercise, enjoying the outdoors and supporting your state park – wins all around. Check into the programs they offer and maybe even volunteer for something. If you don't have a state park nearby, there may be a municipal park – see what is available to you.

Charity Races

If you enjoy the walks for charity, consider doing a 5K or even a bigger race for charity. I have tried this a few times. I finished a half marathon once! This particular race had a full-marathon and also a half-marathon that day. I finished the half at the same time that most people finished the full, but I finished. I have the medal to prove it. The coolest thing about a big race is the time spent preparing for it, which means that you are getting consistent workouts. I am not a good runner – at all. The few times I did a big race, I always made sure to have cab fare safety-pinned inside my shorts in a baggie – just in case. When I did a 10-mile run, I was so slow at the end that the race ambulance actually had to pass me. When I finally got to the end party the only thing left was lemon yogurt – yuck. But, I finished. I have that medal too. I might one day finish a marathon, but that is not high on my goal list. My latest initiative with races is running in vineyards. I discovered that these vineyard runs give you wine afterward. Score!

Golf

I love to play golf. As is the case with running, I'm not a good golfer. If I want to shoot 72, then I need to stop at the 15th hole. I pick up my ball a lot. But hey, all that bending over is calisthenics, right? Now, if you are riding in the cart and sipping mimosas as you go, then you aren't going to be able to count this round of golf as exercise. Probably a great time -- but not exercise.

You should also know that environmentalists don't especially like golf courses. The maintenance of a golf course requires the use of a large amount of water, fertilizers, pesticides, and the consumption of multiple resources. The maintenance of golf courses may also contribute to the pollution of local waterways via storm-water run-off which contains excess nutrients. Or, in the case of water scarcity, they may be taking water away from other uses. Your local golf course likely gets its water from the same source that your household does. The green has to be green, after all. Check into your local courses. They may have enviro-friendly practices and be a part of The United States Golf Association Environmental Stewardship Program. If your local course measures up to your environmental standards, then give it a try. Even if you only go to the driving range to hit a bucket of balls and don't ever actually play a round, it's still exercise and you can still get some new cute outfits.

In and On the Water

I am lucky to live where there is water all around me. If you can get out on the water, then do it. It's good for your soul as well as your body. Even in the winter months, I am in the water. I belong to my local YMCA, which has an indoor pool. I take a class called Deepwater Workout. They also offer Aqua Zumba and have lap lanes as well as an open pool. I bring the kids and we swim. Sometimes we bring a ball and have a catch. If there are enough other kids in the pool, we'll play Marco Polo or Sharks and Minnows. At the end of open swim time, we take a shower in the locker room, put on our jammies, go home and then go to bed. It's awesome. See what is available in your area when the weather is too cold to be on the water outdoors.

Of course, I prefer when the weather warms up and I can get out on the water outside.

I have a SUP (stand up paddle board) that I bought on a layaway plan. I made payments once a month, December through May, and picked it up in time for the nice weather. We have plenty of nice flat water for me to go out on where I live.

The activities of paddlers, which consist of people who kayak, canoe, and stand up paddle board, are tracked by The Outdoor Foundation which was established by the Outdoor Industry Association. They list their mission on their website, "to inspire and grow future generations of outdoor enthusiasts." If you think down the value chain, it makes perfect sense that the companies who manufacture equipment for paddlers have a stake in the preservation of the environment in which their products are used. It stands to reason also that these companies engage in sustainable manufacturing practices, with minimal impact on the environment. The Outdoor Foundation publishes a research report.

Check it out if you are interested in learning more at outdoorindustry.org/participation.

Yoga

My favorite physical activity is yoga. I feel incredibly empowered when I am rocking a warrior pose. Then the next moment, I am completely humbled when I fall out of eagle pose. That's yoga and that's life. I've had instructors say that where you struggle on the mat is where you struggle in life. It's called a "practice" and that's what you do -- practice.

I dig the spiritual aspect of yoga too. Namaste (the spirit in me honors the spirit in you.) I have tried several types of yoga -- Hatha, Vinyasa flow, Ashtanga, and Bikram (where the room is heated). I prefer the boutique yoga studios where someone places an orange-ginger soaked cloth on my forehead during the final resting pose savasana, but my budget prefers the classes at the YMCA. So, I mix it up to please both.

If you have only ever tried one type of yoga class at one type of studio, then you haven't tried yoga. Branch out. Try different things. Your body will thank you. Besides building your muscles and flexibility, yoga is also said to lower your blood pressure and improve your digestion, core strength, circulation, and posture. Plus, you get to buy more cute outfits. I've even combined my love of yoga with my love of SUP (standup paddle board) by taking a SUP yoga class. Don't worry -- you anchor your board before you start into the yoga poses. Try it!

Video games

If you have the gumption and budget to try new things, consider getting interactive video games. If you like a sport or activity on an interactive video game and you can do it fairly well on the video game, then maybe you're ready to try it for real. For example, I have a snowboarding game on Nintendo Wii. This game uses a balance board you stand on in front of your TV so that your moves on the balance board translate to the moves of the character on the screen. In this game, I can stay upright on the snowboard all the way down the hill. I can even pull off cool jumps and board grabs. This does not translate to my real life.

I have a goal, that I have not yet accomplished, to stay upright on a snowboard all the way down the training hill. I have no goals that involve jumps or board grabs, as I prefer to keep my bones together rather than fractured or broken. However, I believe it is a reasonable goal for me to stay upright, not on my butt, down the training hill. I will keep at it. Consider trying something new on a video game, and maybe later, in real life. You don't always have to buy the games to try them. Check your library or second-hand resale store. These places are where I get most of my games.

Play Like a Kid

Do you take your kids to the playground? Do you sit on the bench and watch? If you do, then get up and play. Swing on the monkey bars. Do some pull-ups and leg raises. Swing on the swings. Run. Play. Do your kids like trampoline parks? Do you sit there among the cubbies of sneakers while your kids go out and jump? Do your kids like roller skating or ice skating? Get out there and play along with your kids. Get your behind off the bench. You'll all be happier for it.

Mix it Up

Other fun things to try to include: bike riding, tennis, rock climbing, skiing, Zumba, kick-boxing, etc. Again -- more cute outfits. I take a cardio-kickboxing class at one of the karate studios in my town. It is especially great to go in there after I've had a not-so-great day at the office. Where I work at least, you can't punch people when you might want to – but in my kickboxing class -- yeah, it's on. What do you like to do?

I continually try new things. Sometimes when I try something new that I think that I will like, I end up hating it. Sometimes when I try something new, I am so bad at it that I end up feeling like a total loser. If that happens to you too, it's really okay. What is not okay is to sit on your butt on a bench or a sofa. Just move on and try something else. If you lack inspiration as to what else to try, then make a visit to a retail chain sporting goods store. There are aisles and aisles of things to try. Pick something and go for it.

Yard Work

Do more yard work. If you don't have your own yard then consider helping someone else by working in their yard. Places like nursing homes, senior centers, children's hospitals, State parks, etc. often rely on volunteers to do things like spread mulch, rake leaves, pull weeds and other similar activities. See what is available in your area for volunteer opportunities. You will be helping your body, helping the planet and also helping that organization. You rock.

I love to work in my yard. I love to push the mower. I love to pull weeds. I love to work in my garden. As a single mom, I am happy and grateful to have a yard full of grass to mow and weeds to pull. I put the weeds in the compost pile but I leave the grass clippings in the yard. My grass is thick and lush and I never use commercial chemical fertilizers on my yard or garden. Yardwork is good for your body and the planet. Something cool to put in your yard is a rain garden. You dig this area a little bit lower than the rest of your yard. The point is to give rain water somewhere to collect and pool so it has time to get absorbed into the ground and not runoff your lawn into the street and down the storm drain. When you have runoff like that, the water picks up all kinds of contaminants from the street and hard surfaces that end up in streams, rivers, the ocean, etc. After traveling through your rain garden that has stones and plants that are native to your area, clean filtered water will go to the aquifer.

If you don't know what plants are native to your area, your local big box do-it-yourself store probably has a native plant display in their gardening section. Where I live, the agricultural school of the local university holds an annual native plant sale. Research it. You might be surprised at what you find. You'll have a rain garden that is beautiful and functional; and you did some exercise putting it all together. You've rocked your body and the planet!

PUT GOOD STUFF ON YOUR BODY

Post Yard-Work Bliss

When I'm finished working in my yard, I'm a dirty, sweaty mess, so I get right into the shower. But yardwork days aren't typical days. After I towel off from the shower I apply a deep pore-cleansing mask to my face and neck and a damage-repair mask to my hair. Then it's back into the shower to rinse off. This time after I towel off, I apply a nice, rich body butter and then put on some sweatpants and a T-shirt. Then I chill on the sofa with the remote control and a

glass of wine. I love my spa – I mean yardwork -
- days.

Don't Be an Accidental Polluter

It's encouraging to see natural ingredients
in health and beauty products like the ones I use
on my spa days. But I propose that you ask
yourself some questions like the ones that follow
about the ingredients before you make a
purchase and use these products. Where did
they get the seaweed that they put in the mask?
Are they growing it in a lab somewhere? Or, are
they bottom-trawling the sea floor, tearing up
ecosystems? What exactly did they burn in order
to get the charcoal? What was emitted in the
burning process? Does argan oil really only
come from Morocco? If so, what are the
environmental impacts of shipping it all over the
globe? What exactly are the "botanicals" that the
label lists in these products? "Fragrance" is one
of the most closely held proprietary ingredients

in personal care products, so you are not likely to find out just what exactly is used to make the "fragrance."

My point is for you not to be duped by the promise of "all natural." When I was a child and I tried to tout the righteousness of something as being "all natural," my father scowled, furrowed his brow, and said to me, "Cocaine is all natural. That doesn't make it good for you." While harsh, my father's words were effective. I learned at a young age not to believe the hype; and, to ask my own questions in order to understand what was really going on. The best decisions are informed decisions.

You might be an accidental polluter if you use personal care products with microbeads. Check your scrubs and cleansers. These plastic microbeads go down the drain and into the water supply. Sometimes they are ingested by marine life. Many municipalities have begun to ban their use. What are you washing down the drain? Your skin is your body's biggest organ. What you put on your skin gets absorbed into your body. You are probably conscious about not eating pesticides, but are you absorbing pesticides through your skin care products? Check the labels. Google the names of any ingredients that you don't recognize.

PUT GOOD STUFF
IN YOUR BODY

While moving your body is important, you also have to pay attention to what you eat. You've heard it before – eat local, eat fresh. I have a standing entry on my calendar for lunch hour on Friday to go to the local farmer's market to buy produce.

Community Supported Agriculture

Some areas offer the opportunity to take part in a CSA (Community Supported Agriculture). These programs allow you to join as a member, or buy a share in a local farm. Generally, you pay a certain set fee for your share of the season. Each week, when the farmer's crop is ready to be picked, a box of the weekly produce is set aside for you. In some programs you pick up the box. In other programs the box is dropped off for you. You get freshly picked food directly from the farmer who grew it. The farmer gets financial support from the community to operate the farm. It's a win-win. It can be a cool adventure when you pick up your CSA box. Many times I have picked up an item and wondered "what is this and how the heck do I prepare it?" My farmer included an index card which listed the identity of all of the goodies in the box. If you don't know what it is or how to prepare it, then Google is your friend. If you are not sure if this is available in your area, just type "find a CSA near me" in your internet browser.

Smoothies

Sometimes, your CSA box will give you more of something then you can use right away. I freeze a lot of fruit. You don't have to make banana bread every time your bananas start to get brown spots. Slice and freeze the bananas and then use them in a smoothie later. I do this with most of my fruit. I eat it and use it fresh and then when it starts to turn, I slice it and freeze it. A bag of frozen fruit and a scoop of ice cream is a nice treat, but it's not breakfast. Look up some recipes online. Get a book of smoothie recipes from the library. I use spinach in smoothies a lot. Before you gag, consider that a cup of sliced spinach (no stems in your smoothie please) some sliced strawberries or peaches or mango and some coconut water or passion fruit juice swirled in your blender with some crushed ice makes a delicious breakfast that you can sip on your commute. You're that much closer to 5-a-day (recommended daily serving of fruits and vegetables) and you haven't even gotten to work yet. You can add in some of those super powder mixes (matcha, acai, flax, moringa, chia, etc.) that you get in the health food store too. When you eat what the local farmer is growing, you are rocking your body and the planet.

Buy Local

Your local farmer is likely to be using sustainable farming practices and may be utilizing organic practices. They generally grow a variety of crops on a rotation that is best for the nutrients of their soil. They are not big factory farms with contracts and obligations to big chemical companies. Because the farmers are local, the food they grow is not contributing to transportation pollution, such as greenhouse gas emissions, which contribute to climate change.

Farmscraping

In cities and urban areas, food is being grown in buildings that previously had other lives, perhaps as a warehouse or high-rise. Farmscraping (a farm skyscraper) is where food gets grown vertically so it doesn't take of lot of land space.

You need local farmers just as much as they need you. Where will your food come from if there are no local farmers? I'm not suggesting that you should stop eating imported food. A lot of foods that I love don't grow where I live. What I am suggesting is that you find out what foods grow where you live, find out who is growing it, and find out how you can support these growers. Eating local fruits and vegetables help you to rock your body and the planet.

Local Education Programs

My local high school has an FFA program. FFA is a National Organization for Agricultural Education. The initials come from the original name, Future Farmers of America. The group offers educational opportunities for students in agribusiness, food, plant, and animal sciences. Some schools have sales of the plants they grow in class, including tomatoes and other vegetables and other agricultural products. Some areas have 4H programs. 4H (Head, Heart, Hands and Health) focuses on health, science, agriculture and citizenship programs. Check into what agricultural programs the schools in your area do. You will be supporting the schools, while rocking your body and the planet.

The Local Store

Maybe you don't have a farmer's market, CSA, FFA or 4H program or direct access to locally grown food. You do have a grocery store and it has a produce department. Apples, oranges and bananas are awesome, but branch out and try something new. If you don't know what something is or how to prepare it, then just Google it. I often chuckle in the grocery store check-out line when I have to explain to the clerk what I am buying so that he or she knows how to enter it in the register.

I cook. When I was younger everything that I "cooked" began with a box. Not so anymore. Now my pantry and my refrigerator are stocked with ingredients. You might have heard the advice, "shop the perimeter of the grocery store", because that is where all the fresh stuff is. The pre-packaged preservative-laden chemically-enhanced stuff is usually in the middle aisles. While that may be true, don't throw shade on all the middle aisle stuff. I use a lot of dried beans and legumes in my cooking. Canned crushed tomatoes, olive oil, olives, lots of things that are actually good for your body, can be found in the middle aisles.

Learn to read labels. Don't always cook the same thing. There are recipes everywhere. Facebook, websites, social media, magazines, or if you want to actually hold a cookbook, then go to the library where there are shelves full of cookbooks. You don't have to buy recipes unless you want to. When you find recipes full of vegetables and fruits that you can buy from local growers, you have hit the jackpot!

Plan Ahead

You might be wondering how a single mom with a job, and three kids in travel sports has time to cook. The same skill that allows me to juggle everyone's schedule is how I get it done. Plan ahead. You can wreck your budget and your diet with drive-thru, more on that later, or you can plan ahead. A slow cooker/crockpot can make so much more than mushy stew. (I

have a banging recipe for slow-cooker meatloaf –
it's awesome) Use your slow cooker to prepare
dinner at least twice a week. Pre-assemble the
ingredients for your slow cooker meals and
freeze them in freezer baggies. Write the
directions on the freezer bag with sharpie before
you fill it, for example 8-10 hours on low. In the
morning, when you start the coffee pot, start the
slow cooker. When I have time on the weekends,
usually a Sunday, I'll make a big pot of chili or
some other bean-featured dish. Then I've got a
go-to for lunches and heat-and-eats for the kids
when they get home from school.

You can also prepare foil packs with
things like sausage, cabbage, potato and onion.
The foil packs stack nicely in the fridge so when I
get home from work I just have to fire up the
grill and cook the foil packs right on the grill.
Another quick dinner I love is baked potato
buffet. Microwave some potatoes and then
choose your toppings: chili, broccoli, cheese or

whatever else is in the fridge. Experiment. Eat more produce. I once set a goal for myself to eat salad every day. I tried to do it several times. They say that you have to do something four days in a row in order to make it a habit. I didn't make it. I've found that I can realistically eat salad three times a week. That works for me. See what will work for you.

How Long Will It Stay Fresh?

What makes food shelf-stable? Just how are those middle aisle items able to sit there for so long waiting for you to buy them without refrigeration and without spoilage? Where does that miracle food come from? What happens to it when you eat it? Does it stay in your body as long as it stays on the shelf? Do you wonder these things?

Some research suggests that your body can't process and digest the preservatives so they just get stored inside your body. I hope that if you haven't thought about it before, or if you have thought about it but felt powerless to do anything about it -- that all changes for you now. You have the power! You control what you put into your body. I've heard many conspiracy theories. People like to complain to me that "The Man" is trying to poison them and is messing with the food supply, etc. etc. My response is always the same. "I am happy that you are paying attention to what you are putting into your body. I am happy that you are concerned about what some food manufacturing practices do to human health and the environment. But remember, in a free economy, the consumer has the power. You vote with your dollars. Educate yourself and act accordingly. You have the power to rock your body and the planet."

Make Your Own

There are many benefits to preparing your own food. You know exactly what goes into the meal that you're eating. This is not the case when you buy prepared food in a restaurant, or drive-thru, or convenience store. When my kids were younger, we used to rely on fast food. I wasn't prepared ahead of time. I had to get home from work, pick up the kids, drop off the kids, there was no time to cook dinner so we would just get something on the road. I used to think that the drive-thru was the answer. Then I discovered the selection of healthy choices at the convenience store. They have pre-made salads, fruit cups, protein snacks, boiled eggs, yogurt and veggie snacks in addition to the traditional bags and boxes of snacks. They also have the ability to make you a sandwich or hot meal. If you have a few minutes to get out of the car, go into the convenience store. The choices are better than in the drive-thru.

If you have a few more minutes, go into a grocery store. The stores in my area have a decent selection of ready-to-eat foods, most of which can be eaten in the car just as easily as anything from a fast food drive thru. If you know what you want to pick up and you do the self-checkout, it might not take any longer than the drive-thru line. When you don't have something prepared and ready at home, these are the best choices.

I know how easy it is to take a frozen pizza and have a meal ready in 25 minutes. You can recycle the paperboard box, and depending on where you live, you might be able to recycle the plastic shrink wrap. But it isn't really good for your body, and there isn't really anything inside the box that resembles anything that grows in nature. I know it's a lot to ask of you to give up convenience. So I won't ask you to.

Instead, consider other options for cheap, quick, and easy. "Quick in the now" might be due to "prep work in the past", but really, everything is prepped somewhere. You can have quick food that was prepped in a factory and sealed in a cardboard box, or you can have quick food that was prepped in your kitchen and sealed in food storage containers.

Think about it. Some stores offer fabulous selections of pre-prepped, ready-to-eat healthy foods. By taking this route, you sacrifice cheap, but when you don't have time for prep, the cost for the prepared food may be worth the cost of your time. It's okay if the "work" of the prep is done by someone else.

In my town, we have a BBQ place that does catering as well as table service. I order a small tray of pulled chicken from the catering menu, without sauce. The menu says it serves 12-15 people. I use it all week to make lunches. I put the chicken in salads, wraps, sandwiches, chicken salad, etc. Of course, it can also be heated up for dinners as the restaurant intended. Would something like that work for you and your situation?

Ethnic Foods

When you get stuck about what to cook or get bored with cooking and eating the same old grub all the time, consider different ethnic foods. I find inspiration on the food channel cooking shows.

Recently I was watching a show in the waiting area while having my car serviced. The chef was preparing a dish from Trinidad. I had nothing else to do until my car was done so I entered "Trinidad cookbook" into my internet browser and ended up ordering a bundled set of Caribbean-style cookbooks.

I wasn't always so adventurous. If you aren't used to cooking or trying new things, you can feel overwhelmed. When I was a kid you could tell the day of the week by what Mom put on the dinner table. Monday was chicken. Tuesday was leftovers. Wednesday was spaghetti. Thursday was leftovers. Friday was fish and mac-n-cheese. Saturday was burgers or pizza. Sunday was ham or roast beef. All always prepared the same way. The mother of six children, Mom didn't have time to be adventurous.

I've always liked trying new things. I had spinach for the first time at my friend's house when I was in high school. Her mom was Italian, and she sautéed the spinach in olive oil with garlic. It was fabulous.

When I went to college and got a job, I ate out a lot and it showed. I didn't really learn to cook meals that didn't start with a box until after I had a family. I learned about foods by watching the food shows on TV. The point is that you don't need to worry about what you don't know. Try new things. Try different herbs, spices, fruits, vegetables and ways to cook them. The more the food you eat resembles the way that food grew in nature, the better for your body, and the better for the planet.

The Global Food Supply

The FAO (Food and Agriculture Organization of the United Nations) and the WHO (World Health Organization) monitor the food supply on a global scale. In the United States, there are two authorities that regulate what can be added to food. They are the United States Food & Drug Administration (FDA) and the United States Department of Agriculture (USDA). Both have excellent websites, and both are very good at what they do. The FDA enforces the Federal Food, Drug, and Cosmetic Act with the purpose of protecting consumers. But as the consumer, you need to stay educated.

Factory Farms

As I mentioned before, I'm a fan of CSAs, local farms, orchards and vineyards. Farm-to-table means the food was grown locally. But you should know that "farm fresh" could also be from a factory farm. Basically a factory farm is a big business farm. The farmer produces "product" for food companies (a.k.a. agribusiness) to process, package, and sell to consumers. The farm is a business, so the emphasis is on through-put and profit. Basic economics says that in order for the consumer to buy food cheaply, it needs to be produced/manufactured cheaply. The agribusiness is not going to sell product at a loss, or they wouldn't be in business very long. Good economics makes good sense, so what is the problem?

Factory farming is a term often used by those concerned about animal welfare in the meat and dairy industries. These concerns generally center around animal cruelty. The term is also used in reference to concerns of treating the animals with hormones and steroids. These concerns go beyond the animals to bio-trespass. The concern is that the hormones and steroids given to the animals will accumulate in the bodies of the people who eat them.

How can you know if your food came from a factory farm? You might not be able to find out the names of the farms that grew the food you buy in the store. But, the agribusinesses for which the farms grow the food generally have statements on their websites about their farming and growing practices. Or, if you want a wider range of research, just type the company name and the words "factory farm" into your internet search engine. You can also look at the Business Benchmark on Farm Animal Welfare (BBFAW). They report on hundreds of food companies globally.

Environmental Impact of Factory Farming

I live in the Chesapeake Bay watershed which is a case study for the environmental impact of factory farming. A topographic map of the Chesapeake Bay looks like a lizard with long legs and long tail. At the top of Bay, a.k.a. the Upper Bay the water is fresher, because it comes in primarily from the Susquehanna River. The salinity increases gradually as you move from the upper bay down to the ocean. The Chesapeake Bay has suffered from non-point source pollution from rainwater runoff rich with nutrients from poo from cow farms in Pennsylvania and from chicken farms on the Delmarva Peninsula.

At first it sounds like a simple case of proper poo management. However, there is ongoing debate regarding who owns the poo, and therefore, who exactly is responsible for it. At times, the chicken growers' contracts are written in such a way that the agribusiness (big chicken company) owns the chickens and the feed, and the farmer is responsible to grow the chickens using that certain feed in a prescribed certain way, and then, when the time is right, the chicken company gets their chickens back to be processed.

At no time did the chicken companies make any claim of responsibility for the production waste, ie poo, generated in the process. You may ask "Why not just repurpose the poo? Use it as fertilizer? Sell it as a raw material for some other "product"? Due to variances in consistency of the components, the poo cannot be reliably used as a raw material in other "products".

The farmers have little choice but to stockpile mounds of poo. The rainwater then carries the poo containing nitrogen and phosphorous into the bay. Excess amounts of nitrogen and phosphorous, through processes with algae, take the oxygen out the water so the animals die (eutrophication). Poo is not the only non-point source pollution damaging the Bay, but it is a big problem. Please, one of you smart people reading this, figure out a poo management process and help to save the Bay. Check out the Chesapeake Bay Foundation website at www.cbf.org/.

Aquaculture

We've talked about farming and some environmental impacts of farming on waterways, but did you know that some farmers farm seafood? Aquaculture is a thing. Fisheries management is a big deal. They are tasked with ensuring that fish like tuna, swordfish, marlin, cod, halibut, and flounder aren't being overfished. It stands to reason that some enterprising individuals figured out that they can farm fin fish and shell fish. The last I read, just about half of the seafood being eaten was farmed rather than wild caught. Check out the Monterey Bay Seafood Watch program at wwwseafoodwatch.org/.

Fish Poo Too

If you are buying frozen seafood, take a look at the package and look for claims of sustainability. You should know that aquaculture can also contribute to adverse environmental effects. It's counterintuitive. How can growing fish in the water cause environmental problems? Well, unlike in the wild, the fish are confined to a certain area so their waste accumulates on the bottom of the area where they are contained, and isn't spread out over a large area where they might swim in the wild. Again, it's a problem of poo.

When you pack animals close together it can create an ideal environment for disease and parasites. As with the factory farms on land previously discussed, the farmers may resort to hormones and antibiotics to control these factors, which again, can lead to bio-trespass into the bodies of the people who eat the farmed animals.

For fish in the wild, regulators implement a total allowable catch for a species in an attempt to prevent overfishing. This is typically set to the maximum sustainable yield that is calculated based on a growth model. If you are interested in learning more about fisheries, read some of the research done by Ray Hilborn and publications by the Marine Stewardship Council.

One Vegan Day

Let me propose to you a concept that I call "Vegan Day." A vegan does not eat any animal products. When I first learned about the environmental impacts of animal food production, I felt that I should stop eating animal products, so I've tried to do it - a few times. Giving up dairy is a struggle for me, and I usually don't make it a full two days on a vegan diet. Knowing this about myself, I have adjusted my goal to one that I can realistically do. One day a week I have vegan day. One day a week might not sound like much, but I am talking about leverage points here. If many people took one day a week to be a vegan day, then the impact would be significant. Can you do it?

Yuck Bucket

When considering growing food, the health of soil is important. I have always liked to play in the dirt. My Dad always had a vegetable garden, and we always had a compost pile. Today in my kitchen I have what I lovingly refer to as the "yuck bucket."

In its previous, more glamorous life, my yuck bucket was a 5-gallon ice-cream tub. Today, it collects my organic kitchen scraps. Carrot and potato peels, onion skins, tops of strawberries, ends of celery stalks, avocado skins after I've scooped out the fabulous green flesh, etc. Every couple of days the yuck bucket gets dumped on top of my compost pile by my garden. When I dig up my garden to prep it for planting in the Spring, I mix some compost into the soil a few weeks before I plant that year's vegetables. Composting puts organic matter into the soil.

Healthy Soil

I didn't think too much beyond this until I took a Plant Science class. Healthy soils are needed to grow the food for the growing population, preferably without damaging the soil so that it can continue to feed future generations. Farmers have been trying to produce more food from the same soil for years. Approaches to this include the use of fertilizers, pesticides and genetically modifying crops. Technologies in the 1950s and 1960s allowed farmers to dramatically increase their yields by using pesticides in what is referred to as the Green Revolution.

Every Environmental student reads Rachel Carson's book *Silent Spring,* in which she exposed the dangers of pesticide use, particularly bioaccumulation of DDT, to the world. In the past, some insecticides contained arsenic. Any fields that once received waste water or sludge or industrial areas or mining areas could have heavy metals in the soil. Throughout history, civilizations have thrived and perished based upon their knowledge of the soils that sustained them. My Plant Science class introduced me to the author Jared Diamond. You should check out his books, especially my favorites, *Collapse* and *Dirt*.

Have you thought about where agricultural water comes from? It comes from rivers, lakes and aquifers. Growing food is one of the most water intensive things that we do. So with the same soil, we are trying to grow more food with higher yields that need less water. That's a lot to ask, but what choice do we have? These are the five forming factors of soil: parent material, climate, biota, topography, and time. That parent material can be blown by the wind, or arrive with flood waters, or just have formed where it is. Don't worry, there won't be a quiz, but you should form some understanding of how all these things play a role in the formation of healthy soil, and how healthy soil is important to the growing of food.

Vineyards

Vineyards are some of my favorite places. My favorite ones are the ones where I can pack a picnic, sit on the veranda overlooking the vineyard, and enjoy my picnic with a bottle of their wine. Pure bliss. Vineyards often have cool social events too. The fruit is grown right there on the vine, and then in the wine cellar, it is crafted into the absolute deliciousness that ends up in your glass. More pure bliss.

Vineyards generally utilize organic techniques to grow their grapes. Wineries tend to be environmentally savvy, because climate is a critical factor in the growing of grapes. My affection doesn't stop with wine. I am also a fan of cideries, breweries, and distilleries. All of which depend upon quality agricultural products for their respective crafts. I highly recommend touring a craft brewery or distillery. These people are truly passionate about the use of quality, environmentally friendly ingredients to create their products. I also believe that the best cocktails have fruit and herbs in them. The way that I make my favorite cocktail, the mojito, contains mint leaves and lime, lemon rum, and agave. It's practically a salad.

Well-being on a Budget

Some people have told me that it costs too much to eat healthy food. If that is your position, I suggest you consider how much you pay for your smart phone, or your data plan. I believe that the food you eat to fuel your health is worth as much, if not more, than your phone and your data plan. You need to decide what is right for you.

Sometimes my lunch budget doesn't allow for more than a five dollar fill-up at the drive thru. Consider, though, if you went to the grocery store with that same five dollars. You could buy a whole bag of apples, a fruit and cheese tray, or a crudité platter instead. Always just take a moment and consider your choices to make the best one to rock your body and the planet.

Leftover Buffet

When you develop the habit of preparing food consistently, especially if you cook for more than one person, at some point you will probably have to deal with food waste. Make dinner the night before trash day your *leftover buffet*. Set the table like usual with plates, placemats and silverware, and then put all the containers of leftovers from the fridge on the table. Everyone makes a plate and then takes turns with the microwave. Anything that remains after *leftover buffet* goes out with the garbage the next day, or to the compost pile.

Stone Soup

When I was a kid I read a story called *Stone Soup* by Ann McGovern. It's about a travelling man who convinces a town to pitch in a little something so that at the end he has a fabulous soup to share with all. His contribution? A stone. It's all he has. Individually, each person only had a carrot or a potato, but by adding all of their little somethings together, they made a grand soup. Remember this story when you are looking at the containers in your fridge. Maybe you have just a quarter cup of peas and a half cup of rice from your Chinese take-out. Throw them into a pot with a diced potato, a diced carrot and some chicken stock, and you could have another meal.

Experiment with what you find in your fridge. Add some herbs and spices from your pantry. The first few times you do this it might turn out to be terrible. That's OK. You were going to throw those things out anyway. Eventually, you will make yourself some pretty awesome stone soup.

Of course, you can also start out with the intention of making soup and purposely gather all of the ingredients you will need. You will be amazed at how many more vegetables you incorporate into your diet once you start making yourself a pot of soup at least once a week. Soup is great in a packed lunch, an afterschool snack, TV-watching-snack, etc. Once it has been prepared, soup is the ultimate heat-and-eat food.

Food Festivals

In my town on the third Saturday of August we have the Annual Peach Festival. I absolutely love agricultural festivals. It's community bonding around an agricultural product, heritage, history, community spirit, good food -- what's not to love? Just don't go eating the deep-fried Oreos -- you're totally missing the point if you do. The only downside to big festivals is the amount of trash that results. Festivals tend to specialize in single-use plastics that aren't recycled. Please manage your materials. And don't litter! Nothing drives me crazier than seeing pollution from litter all over the place. Except maybe balloons.

I absolutely hate balloons. Most people don't realize that they are accidentally polluting every time they let a balloon go. Eventually it will come down. Eventually it will end up in the water or the belly of some poor animal. And those lantern festivals -- Ugh! People release their cares and worries with these lanterns and watch them float away. Group littering is what that is.

Of course, not all the food you get at a festival is the agricultural "good stuff." A lot of it is the equivalent of fast food. I love a reuben with curly fries, fried chicken and coleslaw, tacos, and I can't resist that time of year when the green mint milkshakes come out. I won't be a hypocrite and suggest that you banish fast food from your diet. But I urge you to know and accept what you are putting into your body. How much of that food is really food and not artificial sort-of-food? How long will it stay in your body and what effects will it have long-term?

Consider the source of the food. Was the meat factory farmed in a developing country where the land was obtained in a cheap land grab? A land grab is a term to describe a situation when someone, typically from a different location, comes in and obtains land, often inexpensively, who then uses the land for profit without benefitting the locality where the land is located. Was rainforest cleared to make a cow pasture? Were the chickens crowded into a henhouse so that they couldn't move and could only get quickly fat enough to slaughter? The food at fast food places didn't come from a local farm. It wouldn't be so cheap if it did.

Further, fast food is usually packaged up into plastic bags, with plastic utensils. It's paired with a flavored sugar drink with a plastic straw and handed to you through a window while you wait in your running car emitting greenhouse gases. If you are going to indulge, then know and accept what you are doing. Recycle when you're done.

The Last Straw

Skip the straw if you can. I recognize it's easier to skip the straw when you're sitting at a table to eat and not moving in the car. Most people don't realize how harmful straws are to the environment. They seem harmless and they are ubiquitous. The problem with straws is that they don't get recycled. They end up in landfills, in waterways, and inside animals. Plus, they stick around for a long, long time. For the most part, they are completely unnecessary. Most people are physically able to drink without them. You just need to raise your cup to your mouth. I've heard protests from people arguing that when they are in a restaurant they don't want to put their mouth on a cup that someone has used before. Really? Let's think that one through.

In a restaurant, someone else has used the cup or glass before. They have also used the plate and the utensils that you are putting in your mouth. If you don't think that the restaurant where you are eating is clean enough, or the restaurant staff has not thoroughly washed and sanitized the dishes that you are using, then you should probably not eat at that restaurant.

Do you use a straw all the time at home? Probably not. Stop using them when you go out.

Some restaurants are using paper straws. This is a better choice than a plastic straw, but you still probably don't need it. There are some people who carry their own re-usable straws. I don't see it catching on as a trend, but I've seen some that come in cute little carrying cases that attach to your keychain. If you are into re-usable straws then by all means, rock that straw. Just know that you don't need it and that sucking through straws all the time will be put wrinkles on your face around your mouth. #strawssuck

Refill, please

As I am writing this, there are activities in the legislation proposing bans on single-use beverage plastic containers like soft drink bottles. In my experience and studies of environmental policy, bans work best when alternatives are proposed. I am not seeing anything being proposed as substitutes to these single use plastics so we'll see where these proposals end up.

In the meantime, don't wait for the government to tell you what to do. The liquids in those single-use plastic beverage containers are probably not something that you really want to put into your body anyway -- read the ingredients. Get yourself a reusable bottle. Fill the bottle with water and add some produce to flavor it. Citrus fruits are a popular choice. So are herbs like mint, thyme, and basil. Also, melon and cucumber can be nice. Experiment and see what you like. Refill a bottle and drink a lot of water.

How About a Nice Cup of Tea?

If water is just too plain and boring for you, then drink tea. You can drink it Queen-style, brewed hot in fancy china cups. You can sip it in a mug with lemon and honey. You can brew it and ice it or add fruits to it. The possibilities are endless. I am talking about the tea leaves you brew by steeping in how water, not the instant powder in the canister. In my pantry right now I have, Green Tea, Black Tea with Jasmine, Chamomile, Ginger Twist, Chai, Oolong, and Pu'erh teas.

Tea has many health benefits. Do a Google search on what type of tea you should drink for whatever ails you. You can grow your own tea at home or choose from the selection on the shelves at the store, grown by professional farmers. As with any type of farming, you will want to be sure your tea is farmed sustainably; and if you buy tea in bags, find out what material the bag is made of. If you buy a particular brand, the company website might have information on the environmental efforts they utilize in producing the tea for you. In some cases, the workers rely on the land-owner not just for the job, but also for housing and healthcare, too. After you have enjoyed your sustainably and ethically grown tea, remember that you can add your used tea bags to your compost instead of throwing them in your trash can. You can also add your used tea bags to your fire pit to repel mosquitos.

One Word: Plastics

Plastic doesn't go away. It can break down, but it doesn't go away. Do you know how much plastic you use each day? Run an experiment for a few days and take note of how much plastic you use. There isn't much that you can do about the plastic that's used in the structure of your car or transportation each day. Not much you can do about the amount of plastic in the structures where you work, live, and go to school.

But what about the things that you can control, like the food you eat and how it is packaged, prepared, served and stored? How much plastic is used? Is that plastic recycled?

There are multiple studies about the migration of chemical components into food from packaging. There are several government agencies that look after the safety of food and food packaging materials globally. With very few exceptions (such as a certain frozen meat-lover lasagna in a red box), I don't microwave food in plastic containers. Use glass and ceramic containers instead.

Are your cleaning supplies and your personal care products packaged in plastic? Do you recycle it? Who is creating the demand for such secure packaging of socks? Getting the plastic tags out without putting holes in the socks is an unnecessary struggle. Plastic is a great material. It is everywhere because it performs its function beautifully. But it needs to be managed well. That management is the job of the people who use it. So manage your plastic well.

Re-usable Bags

Plastic bag pollution is so ubiquitous that it is used as figurative language in pop songs. You know the Katy Perry song *Firework*, "Do you ever feel like a plastic bag? Drifting on the wind, wanting to start again?" Keep re-usable grocery bags in the trunk of your car. When you go to the grocery store take them inside with you in the cart. When it comes time to bag up your groceries, put the purchases into the bags you brought, not the store plastic bags. Sometimes, you buy more stuff than will fit into your bags and you have to use some store plastic bags – it happens.

My local municipality won't take the store plastic bags in my recycle bin, so, I re-purpose them. These bags become the trash bags in my small waste baskets. These bags are the recipients of the clumps when the cat boxes get cleaned out. When I reach the point of having a bag full of bags, that bag gets tossed into the trunk of my car and goes to the grocery store with me. My grocery store has a box in the entry way where they collect back the empty bags for recycling. Does your grocery store take bags back? Some large department stores accept them too. See what is available in your area.

Sustainable Buildings

As I said before, you don't have much control over the plastic materials used in the construction of the buildings you enter. The United States Green Building Council (USGBC) has developed LEED ® (Leadership in Energy and Environmental Design™). A significant amount of greenhouse gases are emitted by buildings and by people commuting back and forth to the buildings. USGBC certifies buildings as green buildings based upon sustainable measures used to build, maintain and operate those buildings. They look at the efficiency of water and energy use, how people get to the building, what materials were used to construct and decorate the building, location of the building, and the indoor environment. Buildings that achieve this certification usually display a plaque describing the achievement. Look for it in the buildings you visit.

The manufacture and use of sustainable products in commercial buildings is a market-driven initiative. That means that you, the consumer, have influence. Even for your home there are carpets and countertops made with recycled contents. There is porcelain made from recycled toilets, tubs and sinks. You decide the sustainable practices of manufacturers by what you buy and the price that you pay for what you buy.

Storm Drain Debris

Are there grates over the storm drains where you live or can trash get down in them?

Do you know where the water goes once it goes down the storm drain? Many times it does not go to a waste water treatment plant but instead goes straight to a waterway. A lot of pollutants and plastics get into streams, rivers, and oceans that way. Most people don't realize that anything that can be moved by the wind will likely end up in the water. Marine debris is such a big thing that NOAA (National Oceanic and Atmospheric Administration) has a Marine Debris Tracker app for your phone. They encourage us all to report on the app what trash we picked up at what location which helps them with their statistics.

The ocean is big. There used to be a saying, thankfully people don't say it anymore, "the solution to pollution is dilution". People actually used to think that they could just flush away their issues. Where is "away" anyway? The official term is Assimilative Capacity. Take note of the second word in the term. Capacity.

All things can only handle so much before they reach the point of no return and get ruined. This is critical, considering the ocean supports all life on planet Earth.

According to the Ocean Conservancy, the deadliest pieces of ocean trash are fishing gear, plastic bags, balloons, cigarette butts, and bottle caps. Seventy percent of the Earth is covered by water. So when you release a balloon into the air, there is a seventy percent chance that it will come down in water. Derelict fishing gear a.k.a. "ghost gear," such as nets, crab pots and fishing traps, is a problem that you might not recognize. Fishermen don't want to lose their stuff, but they do. All of this plastic circulates in the ocean in the gyres, the Pacific Ocean garbage patch, the Gulf Stream, California Current, and the other currents. It is a global problem. The Ocean Plastics Charter was adopted on June 9, 2018 by five of the G7 member nations. I can't wait to see what the outcome will be.

Where's the Well?

Our planet is mostly water. Our bodies are mostly water. So, how are most people so disconnected from water? Do you think about water any other time besides when you turn on the faucet? Do you know where your water comes from? What aquifer is the source of your water? What waste water treatment plant manages your water? What watershed do you live in? Do you know? How polluted are the creeks, streams, rivers and lakes in your area? These are important things to know and monitor as these affect the quality of the water that you need to survive. Like Ben Franklin said, "You know the worth of water when the well runs dry."

Use Less

If you haven't already, watch the Buzzfeed video on YouTube about how much water you use every day. Think about your daily routine and try ways of using less water. Little changes can make a difference. An easy way to keep clear in your mind what potable water is — break down the word like this: potable water is water that you are *able* to put in a *pot* to cook your food. I don't have a lot of counter space in my kitchen so I store the water bottles in a wine rack. Are your appliances and plumbing fixtures water efficient? There is money as well as water to be saved if they are not. Look into the EPA Water Sense program. On their website they list products as well as tips and tools to help you to conserve water. Additionally, The United States Geological Survey compiles data on water use in the US which is available for you on their website. You can compare your water use to see how close you are to the average.

How much electricity do you use? This is another case where being a little more conservative can save you some money while helping the environment. Can you go a few degrees lower or higher on your thermostat? How much TV do you watch? Are you moving while you watch TV? You can be lifting weights, doing leg raises, squats, standing on a balance board, all while watching TV. Don't always use the food processor. Use your muscles and chop some fresh produce on those nights when you're not in such a hurry to get dinner on the table. Do you need to have so many lights on all the time? Have you considered alternative energy? Is it available where you live? In many cases solar panels are worth the investment to have them installed. How much insulation do you have in your home? Does your municipality have an option to purchase green power?

Climate Change and Sea Level Rise

If you live in a land-locked area then you might not think too much about sea level rise. I'm a coastal girl so I think about sea level rise a lot. One particular strip of land where I like to spend time is only a mile wide. One side is ocean and the other side is bay. Some predict that in about a century or so, that strip of land is going to be under water. I tell my kids to enjoy that strip of land as much as they can while it's still here. You might have guessed that this particular strip of land is a beach town. It is built up to the max. Everybody wants to go there. It's beauty and attraction will cause it's death. Sad but true.

I suspected that most people think that there isn't anything that can be done about sea level rise. My suspicion was confirmed when I heard the song, *"Trip Around the Sun"* by Kenny Chesney. It starts out like this, "Well they say the sea is rising, well that's alright with me. 'Cause there ain't no other place than on the sea I'd rather be. ... There ain't nothin we can do about the whole thing anyway." I challenge you to educate yourself about salt marshes, wetlands, and mangroves. These are natural defenses along the coasts. In addition to providing habitat, they protect against storm surge and erosion. That is, if we don't destroy them. We must resist taking them out to build up hotels and entertainment venues.

Conservation Economics and Valuation of Ecosystems is not just a coastal problem. All of you land-locked people, think about it for a minute, where do you suppose that all of us coastal people are going to go? We're not going down to live with Sponge Bob. We're moving inland. We're coming to your towns. And we're bringing our surfboards with us. All kidding aside, there are whole countries, often referred to as the Small Island States, that are in jeopardy of disappearing. All of these people will become what is called Environmental Refugees. Where will they go?

Two Degrees

The United Nations Framework Convention on Climate Change is an environmental treaty that came about at UNCED (The United Nations Conference on the Environment and Development) UNCED is also known as the Earth Summit and it took place back in 1992. It focused on greenhouse gas emissions and climate change. In 1988, the Intergovernmental Panel on Climate Change (IPCC) was established of climate scientists who have been studying the Earth's climate ever since. IPCC issued their first report in 1990, which stated that the world has been warming and that future warming seemed likely. As a result governments are attempting to work together to keep the warming below two degrees Celsius above pre-industrial levels.

I've been asked by people who don't understand climate change what the big deal is about two degrees. If you think about two degrees like going from 75 degrees to 77 degrees still makes for great picnic weather, then I can see how you are missing the point. You have to look at the big picture and the long-term effects. Think about two degrees being the difference that means the snow won't form on the mountain tops in winter. So there isn't snow to melt in spring. So there isn't water running down the mountain to water the crops. So the people that live at the bottom of the mountain can't grow their crops and don't have enough to eat.

Think about two degrees meaning that some of the glacier ice melts. Where does the water go? Into the ocean. What happens when you put melted ice into a full glass? The liquid spills over the edge. In the ocean that spilling over equals sea level rise. Think about two degrees meaning the ocean is getting warmer. Warmer seas mean more powerful storms. It means storage of carbon dioxide in the ocean which means acidification.

Some scientists are suggesting that the global temperature will increase not two but four degrees above pre-industrial levels in the next century. What effects might that cause? Climate change affects weather, which affects rain, which affects drought, which affects soil, which affects food, which affects life.

The Bottom Line:
Be an Educated Consumer

Environmental and natural resource economics are all about externalities. Government comes in when markets fail to be efficient on their own. You, my readers, are the market. Choices. You have the power to make impactful choices.

For example, choose a paper towel over an air dryer in a restroom. Why? Trees are a renewable resource. The coal that was burned to create the electricity to run that "air" dryer is not renewable, and when burned, emits greenhouse gases that contribute to climate change. Even when you factor in the water consumed to produce the paper towels, and maybe the air dryer's electricity was generated via a solar or wind power, in the end, the paper towel is a better environmental choice for me. I'm not suggesting that everyone needs to know how to calculate an environmental economic analysis of scenarios (although that would be awesome). I am suggesting that you make a habit of learning more.

Be an educated consumer. The market needs to supply what consumers want. If you want to continue to live, then you are going to have to eat. What's good for the planet and what's good for your body are pretty much the same. Because really, the planet and your body are both made out of the same stuff. Love them both.

REFERENCES

BBFAW | Business Benchmark - A benchmark on farm animal welfare. "BBFAW 2017 Report Now Published." BBFAW, www.bbfaw.com/.

Carson, Rachel. *Silent Spring*. Penguin Books, in Association with Hamish Hamilton, 2015.

Chesapeake Bay Foundation: Homepage. Chesapeake Bay Foundation, www.cbf.org/.

Chesney, Kenny, *Trip Around the Sun*, Cosmic Hallelujah Album, Blue Chair Records 2016

Diamond, Jared M. *Collapse: How Societies Choose to Fail or Survive*. Penguin Books, 2011.

Diamond, Jared M. Dirt: The Erosion of Civilizations. Penguin Books, 2008.

Hilborn, Ray."*Ray Hilborn's Web Site*, rayhblog.wordpress.com/.

IPCC - Intergovernmental Panel on Climate Change. *AR4 SYR Synthesis Report Summary for Policymakers - 2 Causes of Change*, www.ipcc.ch/.

Marine Debris Tracker - NOAA Marine Debris Program, dianna.parker. "Marine Debris Tracker | OR&R's Marine Debris Program." Dianna.parker, 10 July 2013, marinedebris.noaa.gov/partnerships/marine-debris-tracker.

Marine Stewardship Council: MSC home, "MSC Home | Marine Stewardship Council." Purse Seine - Marine Stewardship Council, www.msc.org/.

McGovern, Ann, and Winslow Pels.*Stone Soup*. Paw Prints, 2009.

Ocean Conservancy, "Ocean Conservancy."Ocean Conservancy, oceanconservancy.org/.

OCEAN PLASTICS CHARTER, https://g7.gc.ca/wp-content/uploads/2018/06/OceanPlasticsCharter

.pdf, "Sommet Du G7 De 2018 | 2018 G7
Summit."Sommet Du G7 – G7 Summit,
g7.gc.ca/.

Outdoor Foundation. *Outdoor Industry
Association*, outdoorindustry.org/participation/.

Perry, Katy, *Firework*, Teenage Dream Album,
Capitol Records 2010

Running Events in Delaware, Pennsylvania &
Maryland. *Races2Run*, www.races2run.com/.

Seafood Watch - Official Site of the Monterey Bay
Aquarium's Sustainable Seafood Program.
*Fishing and Farming Methods from the Seafood
Watch Program at the Monterey Bay Aquarium,*
www.seafoodwatch.org/.

UNFCCC. United Nations Framework
Convention on Climate Change. *UNFCCC,*
unfccc.int/.

United States Green Building Council homepage
| USGBC, "USGBC Homepage | USGBC." LEED
| USGBC, new.usgbc.org/.

U.S. Geological Survey. www.usgs.gov/.

USGA and Sustainability. USGA,
www.usga.org/course-care/usga-sustainability.html.

WaterSense. *EPA*, Environmental Protection
Agency, www.epa.gov/watersense.

YMCA of the USA: the Y. The Y,
www.ymca.net/index.php.